Methadone Maintenance Treatment

Recommendations for Enhancing Pharmacy Services

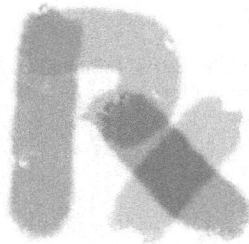

Pearl Isaac and Beth Sproule
for the Working Advisory Panel

camh

Centre for Addiction and Mental Health
Centre de toxicomanie et de santé mentale

Library and Archives Canada Cataloguing in Publication

Isaac, Pearl
  Methadone maintenance treatment : recommendations for enhancing pharmacy services / Pearl Isaac and Beth Sproule, for the working advisory panel.

Includes bibliographical references.
Also available in electronic format.
ISBN 978-1-77052-302-9

  1. Methadone maintenance—Ontario. 2. Pharmacist and patient—Ontario.
3. Pharmacy—Ontario. I. Sproule, Beth II. Centre for Addiction and Mental Health III. Title.

RC568.M4I82 2009   616.86'32061   C2009-904555-9

ISBN: 978-1-77052-302-9 (PRINT)
ISBN: 978-1-77052-304-3 (HTML)
ISBN: 978-1-77052-303-6 (PDF)
ISBN: 978-1-77052-305-0 (ePUB)

This publication may be available in other formats. For information about alternate formats or other CAMH publications, or to place an order, please contact Sales and Distribution:

Toll-free: 1 800 661-1111
Toronto: 416 595-6059
E-mail: publications@camh.net
Online store: http://store.camh.net
Website: www.camh.net

CAMH acknowledges the financial support of the Government of Ontario. The views expressed are the views of the authors and do not necessarily reflect those of the Government of Ontario.

This book was produced by:
Development: Lynn Schellenberg Editorial Services
Editorial: Kelly Coleman, CAMH
Design: Nancy Leung, CAMH
Print production: Chris Harris, CAMH
Typesetting: TC Communications Express

4049 / 10-2009 / PZ170

CONTENTS

ACKNOWLEDGMENTS

Members of the Working Advisory Panel

Pearl Isaac, RPh, BScPhm
Pharmacist, Department of Pharmaceutical Services, CAMH
Lecturer (Status), Faculty of Pharmacy, University of Toronto

Beth Sproule, RPh, BScPhm, PharmD
Advanced Practice Pharmacist / Clinician Scientist,
Department of Pharmaceutical Services, CAMH
Assistant Professor, Faculty of Pharmacy, University of Toronto

Nicole Balan, RPh, BScPhm, MBA, MEd
Manager, Pharmacy Practice Programs
Ontario College of Pharmacists

Carla Beaton, RPh, BScPhm, CGP, FASCP
Regional Director of Operations
Medical Pharmacies Group, Ontario

Geri Dart, RPh, BScPhm
Pharmacist, Peterborough, Ontario

Maja Gavrilovic, RPh, BScPhm, ACPR
Pharmacist, Department of Pharmaceutical Services, CAMH

Eva Janecek, RPh, BScPhm
Pharmacist, Department of Pharmaceutical Services, CAMH
Lecturer (Status), Faculty of Pharmacy, University of Toronto

Anne Kalvik, RPh, BScPhm
Pharmacist, Department of Pharmaceutical Services, CAMH
Lecturer (Status), Faculty of Pharmacy, University of Toronto

Catherine Kelley, RPh, BScPhm
Pharmacist, Toronto West Detention Centre
Ministry of Community Safety and Correctional Services

Satinder Sanghera, RPh, BScPhm
Pharmacy Manager, Scarborough General Hospital Rexall Pharmacy

Other advisors
The authors thanks Betty Dondertman, Manager, Education Services, CAMH, for her input and support during the development of this guide.

Research assistance
The panel thanks Sheila Lacroix, BSc, MLS, Library Coordinator, CAMH Library, for her assistance with the literature search.

Stakeholder reviewers
The authors appreciate the time and care generously given by the reviewers during the external review process.

Christina Cella, RPh, BSc Hons, BScPhm, ACPR
Staff Pharmacist, Quinte Healthcare Corporation, Belleville
President-Elect, Ontario Branch, Canadian Society of Hospital Pharmacists

Iris Greenwald, MD, CCFP, MRO

Susan Halasi, MScPhm
Drug Information Pharmacist, Drug Information and Research Centre, Ontario Pharmacists' Association

Agnes Kwasnicka, MSc, MD, CCFP
Staff physician, Addiction Medicine Services, CAMH

Anne Resnick, RPh, BScPhm
Director, Professional Practice, Ontario College of Pharmacists

Carol Strike, PhD
Senior Scientist, Health Systems Research and Consulting Unit, CAMH

Kate Tschakovsky, MSW, RSW
Clinical Social Worker, Schizophrenia Program, CAMH

FOREWORD

In Ontario, there is a growing problem with opioid addiction, and the majority of people who are using opioids are using prescription medications. Methadone maintenance treatment (MMT) has been proven to be medically effective in helping to stabilize the lives of people wrestling with the difficulties associated with opioid addiction. Within the treatment team, the pharmacist is the only member to see the MMT client every day. This ongoing professional relationship can provide support to the client and contribute to the positive changes that he or she experiences through treatment.

This guide has been developed to offer support to the pharmacist. The dispensing of methadone is unlike any other service provided by the pharmacist and involves special systems and services. The authors make a series of recommendations on ways to encourage pharmacists to provide methadone services, to make service more respectful of and responsive to client needs, to improve the education of pharmacist students and those already practising, and to strengthen interprofessional relationships among the MMT primary care team. This document goes further to suggest ways in which decision-makers at the service and system level may enhance pharmacy services and support pharmacists in their front-line care of MMT clients.

The guide was developed as part of the CAMH OpiATE Project. That Project was funded by the Ministry of Health and Long-Term Care following the release of the report of the Methadone Maintenance Treatment Practices Task Force in the summer of 2007. The Task Force made 26 recommendations in its report, several directed specifically to CAMH.

The Opiate Project's objectives were:

1. To develop sustainable biopsychosocial treatment models for people with opioid dependence by engaging communities to increase awareness of the benefits of treatment for opioid dependence
2. To raise awareness about issues related to opioid dependence and reduce stigma and marginalization of addiction clients
3. To expand training and professional supports, including the development of a certificate program in opioid addiction for nurses, physicians, pharmacists, case managers and counsellors.

The Opiate Project has focused on developing resources (including this guide) to provide information for the public and support professionals who provide treatment. More information about these resources can be found on the website MethadoneSavesLives.ca.

Christine Bois
Opiate Project Manager
CAMH, Ottawa

Background

Introduction

The problem of opioid addiction appears to be growing in Ontario, and is primarily associated with pharmaceutical opioid products rather than heroin. Methadone is an effective treatment for opioid addiction that has been used in Ontario for decades. For many Ontarians struggling with opioid addiction, methadone maintenance treatment (MMT) could save their lives. However, methadone has a unique pharmacological profile that requires specialized knowledge and procedures to ensure its safe use. Pharmacists are at the front line of ensuring the safe and effective use of methadone.

The Centre for Addiction and Mental Health (CAMH) has offered multi-disciplinary training for many years to professionals providing MMT services. In conjunction with this training a comprehensive manual was developed for pharmacists to use in their everyday practice. The current edition, entitled *Methadone Maintenance: A Pharmacist's Guide to Treatment* (Isaac et al., 2004), is a required resource for all pharmacies dispensing methadone in Ontario. A revised edition is now being prepared. The revision will include the other available treatment for opioid addiction—buprenorphine—and will take the form of a best practice guide with clearly delineated recommendations.

During the revision process, the authors determined that there were system-level matters that, if addressed, could significantly enhance the provision of MMT pharmacy services in Ontario. To that end, CAMH decided to develop another, complementary guide, one that could make specific recommendations—outside the scope of the best practice guide, and related to key selected areas of pharmacy MMT services—that would, ultimately, support individual pharmacists in providing safe and effective client care.

The outcome of that decision is the book you have before you. It can be used in a number of ways:

- Pharmacy managers can use it to review how they currently deliver services and identify how they might improve the services they deliver to MMT clients.
- Providers of community health care can use it to think about working with pharmacists to improve interprofessional collaboration and to find additional ways to make pharmacy services more accessible to MMT clients.
- Research and scientific groups can use the recommendations on research priorities as a guide to areas of future study.
- Educators in pharmacy programs can use it to ensure that educational programs reflect best practice in providing pharmaceutical care to clients in MMT.
- Professional regulatory bodies (such as the Ontario College of Pharmacists) can use it to stimulate discussion and introduce change into the requirements for training and evaluation of their members providing MMT services.
- The Ontario Ministry of Health and Long-Term Care and the province's Local Health Integration Networks can use this guide to enhance their understanding of the role of pharmacists and pharmacy services in MMT and to inform decisions about increased or ongoing service and funding.

By working together, these groups can ensure that pharmacy services continue to be enhanced as part of providing optimal care to MMT clients.

About this guide

The purpose of this guide is to identify areas of pharmacy service in methadone maintenance treatment in Ontario that could be enhanced at either the pharmacy or system level. Accordingly, it addresses issues beyond best practice by the individual pharmacist, making recommendations related to the pharmacy environment, pharmacist education programs, accessibility of pharmacy services and research needs. The target audience is pharmacy managers and corporate executives, the Ontario College of Pharmacists, pharmacy educational institutions, research scientists, professional pharmacy organizations and the government. In addition, there are recommendations related to interprofessional collaboration and addressed to other members of the practice team and to the organizations that represent or employ them.

Part I of this guide contains background information, including the processes the panel used to develop the recommendations.

The recommendations in Part II are the core of this guide. They are presented first in summary form, then individually with the supporting research and discussion. Various findings and quotes from the client consultation process (described below) provide the clients' perspectives on pharmacy services in MMT in a selection of communities.

This document is not intended to be a comprehensive primer or best practice guide on MMT for pharmacists. Its recommendations are intended to support best practices by pharmacists at the pharmacy or system level. *Methadone Maintenance: A Pharmacist's Guide to Treatment* (Isaac et al., 2004), now undergoing revision for a new edition, is an important reference for practising pharmacists who dispense methadone, and is available from CAMH.

Overview of the development process

WORKING ADVISORY PANEL

The panel members were selected based on their experiences with MMT services and to represent a variety of practice settings (community pharmacy, hospital practice, long-term care facilities, correctional facilities, specialty addictions facility) from sites across Ontario.

GUIDING QUESTIONS

The members of the panel agreed on the scope and purpose of the document and on four questions that would guide their investigation:

1. What knowledge and skills and attitudes do pharmacists need to provide optimal MMT services safely to opioid-dependent clients?
2. What is required in the pharmacy practice environment to ensure optimal MMT services?
3. What can MMT clients expect from the care they receive from pharmacists and pharmacy practice sites?
4. What is needed to ensure that MMT pharmacy services are available across Ontario?

Once the panel established the parameters of the project, it proceeded to conduct the literature search and evaluation and then to draft the recommendations.

LITERATURE SEARCH AND EVALUATION STRATEGY

The literature review strategy included three steps. The first, a literature review conducted by Reference Services, CAMH Library, searched three core databases for literature on addiction and substance misuse from different discipline perspectives:

- MEDLINE (National Library of Medicine)
- CINAHL (Cumulative Index to Nursing and Allied Health Literature, EBSCO Publishing)
- PsycINFO (American Psychological Association)

The searches were conducted in March 2009 for literature published in the last 15 years. The databases were searched separately, to take advantage of the unique and useful indexing each offers.

See Table 1 for the key words and search strategies used in the individual database searches.

TABLE 1
Key words and search strategies

PsyCINFO
• Run on the 1987 – present database segment

Pharmacists (SH) *or* Pharmacy Service* (ti,kp) *or*
Pharmacies (ti,kp)
and
Drug Abuse Exp (SH) *or* Intravenous Drug Usage (SH) *or* Drug
Rehabilitation Exp (SH) *or* Alcohol Abuse Exp (SH) *or* Drug
Addiction (SH) *or* Drug Dependency (SH) *or* Drug Overdoses (SH)
or Polydrug Abuse (SH)

MEDLINE
• Run 1994 to present

Pharmacists (SH) *or* Education, Pharmacy (SH) *or* Pharmaceutical
Services (SH)
and
Substance-Related Disorders Exp (SH)

• In-process and other non-indexed citations (2008 to present)

Pharmacist* *or* Pharmacy *or* Pharmacies
and
Various drug and alcohol terms, including specific drugs:
Cocaine, Opioids, Opiates, etc. (Results were manually filtered
for relevance, as key word searching results in low specificity.
Nine records were selected.)

CINAHL
• Cumulative Index to Nursing and Allied Health Literature

Pharmacists (SH) *or* Pharmacist Attitudes (SH) *or* Pharmacy
Service (SH) *or* Education, Pharmacy (SH)
and
Substance Use Disorders Exp (SH) *or* Substance Abuse Exp (SH)
or Substance Abusers (SH) *or* Intravenous Drug Users (SH)

---

* = truncation symbol, to allow retrieval of words with variant endings; SH = subject
heading; ti = key word(s) in title; kp = key word in key phrase; Exp = explode (i.e., the
SH and its more narrow SHs are searched for using the Boolean operator "or". For
example, the SH Substance-Related Disorders has 11 more narrow headings, among
them Substance Abuse, Intravenous, Alcohol-Related Disorders (which has 4 more
narrow terms including Alcoholism) and Opioid-Related Disorders; an exploded
search includes all of the narrower subject headings.

After duplicate articles were removed, 62 retrieved publications were evaluated for inclusion. A pharmacist experienced in the field of substance abuse and methadone treatment reviewed articles for relevance. Articles published in peer-reviewed journals and specifically related to MMT were considered.

During the second step, the authors conducted a hand search of literature from the reference lists of publications found in the original literature search as well as of other current resources they were alerted to through database subscription services available to the CAMH Pharmacy team. The third step of the literature review strategy was to conduct a search of the World Wide Web using the search engine Google, to identify grey literature and complementary material such as publications and data from established programs and initiatives, provincial colleges of pharmacy, professional organizations and associations, faculties of pharmacy, and government organizations and ministries.

There were no randomized control studies found. Most studies were surveys, and those with large sample sizes and adequate response rates were considered for inclusion. Those selected included a description of the rationale for study, methodology, results, discussion, limitations, and recommendations for further research. There was very limited research available pertaining specifically to pharmacy services in Ontario and Canada. Most of the pharmacy-based research available was from the United Kingdom or Australia. Because there were very few studies from the United States, the panel included descriptive pilot studies of pharmacy practice in that country.

The panel also reviewed MMT guidelines from various provincial associations and colleges of pharmacy, as well as from other stakeholder groups. In topic areas where there was no other research available, general guidelines were included if they described the methods used for guideline development and where it was clear they were developed through a consensus process. Publications in the area of pharmacist education on substance abuse pre- and post-licensure were also included. Publications that represented clients' views on pharmacy service in MMT and publications dealing with attitudes and practices of MMT pharmacy providers, including the education of pharmacists in these areas, were considered as well.

Data from the selected documents was extracted and summarized. For research studies, the summaries included the type of study, the number and description of subjects, the objectives of the study, the primary outcome and other relevant outcomes, and an assessment of the strengths and weaknesses of the study.

FORMULATION OF RECOMMENDATIONS

Key themes identified from the literature review were organized according to the four guiding questions (page 4) and a subgroup of the panel drafted preliminary recommendations organized by these themes. The resulting preliminary document was sent to all panel members for review; two panel meetings followed at CAMH, Toronto, in May 2009, to discuss and come to group consensus on the recommendations. On the basis of these discussions and consultations, the subgroup revised the draft manuscript. The revised document was sent to external stakeholder reviewers in June 2009. Their comments and feedback suggested further refinements, which the authors incorporated into the final document.

CLASSIFICATION OF RECOMMENDATIONS

Recommendations are classified based on the level of evidence available to support them, as described in Table 2. In the absence of controlled studies, the recommendations in this guide are primarily classified as either Level III or IV.

TABLE 2
Levels of evidence

LEVELS	EVIDENCE
Ia	Evidence obtained from meta-analysis or systematic review of randomized control trials
Ib	Evidence obtained from at least one randomized control trial
IIa	Evidence obtained from at least one well-designed, controlled study without randomization
IIb	Evidence obtained from at least one other type of well-designed, quasi-experimental study without randomization
III	Evidence obtained from well-designed, non-experimental descriptive studies, such as comparative studies, co-relational studies and case studies
IV	Evidence obtained from expert committees, reports, opinions and/or clinical experiences of respected authorities

CLIENT CONSULTATION

A series of interviews with MMT clients* in Ontario contributed another component to this book's development. A client consultation was undertaken in 2008 by an experienced clinical social worker to document clients' experiences and views of pharmacies and case management during their methadone treatment in communities in Ontario. The purpose of the

---

* CAMH prefers the term "client" over "patient" but to reflect the usage and context of sources cited the terms are used interchangeably in this document.

consultation was explained and clients were invited to give their feedback, through a brief, structured interview, on what worked well at the sites where they received their methadone and what changes they would like to see. Although this consultation process focused on both case management and pharmacy, this guide will focus on the pharmacy experiences only.*

Twelve different methadone programs and providers in seven communities asked for client volunteers to participate in the interviews about their experiences with MMT. These communities included four under-serviced, high-need communities identified in the OPiATE Project and a small pilot group in Toronto.

Interviews with 30 women and 39 men, who ranged in age from 19 to 60, were conducted. The majority of the women were in the 21-to-30-year-old category and the majority of men were in the 31-to-40-year-old category.

All of the clients consulted were receiving MMT at the time of their interviews. Most had been on methadone for either under two years (the largest percentage of clients interviewed) or for over five years (the second-largest percentage of those interviewed).

The majority of the clients involved in this consultation (86 per cent) received their treatment at clinics that had multiple services on-site, such as urine drug screening, case management and nursing.

Interviews were one-on-one, lasted about 25 minutes and used a combination of structured and open-ended questions. Clients were paid $20 for their time.

This consultation was not a research study, and its application to the general population of MMT clients in Ontario is limited. It does, however, provide a record of some client concerns and thoughts regarding their experiences with pharmacy services in MMT. Their responses contribute an important perspective to this guide on the subject of pharmacy recommendations, through quotations from the interviews and consultation findings.

* See K. Tschakovsky (2009), *Methadone Maintenance Treatment: Best Practices in Case Management,* Toronto: CAMH, for more of this consultation's findings on clients' experiences in MMT.

PART II

Recommendations and discussion

Summary of recommendations

Please see Table 2 on page 8 for an explanation of the levels of evidence used to classify recommendations.

INTERPROFESSIONAL COLLABORATION AND COMMUNICATION

These recommendations address the second and third questions posed by the panel at the beginning of the development process:

- What is required in the pharmacy practice environment to ensure optimal MMT services?
- What can MMT clients expect from the care they receive from pharmacists and pharmacy practice sites?

The panel recommends that:
1. MMT programs and methadone prescribers recognize the role of pharmacists in collaborative care and this role's impact on their mutual clients' treatment. Specifically, the College of Physicians and Surgeons of Ontario should emphasize in its *Methadone Maintenance Guidelines* the importance of collaboration and regular communication with the pharmacist and their impact on patient care and safety. [IV]

2. Prescribing physicians and MMT programs establish and then maintain communication with community pharmacists regarding client treatment plans and progress. [IV] In particular, the panel recommends that:

 a. At the outset of MMT, the prescribing physician initiate contact and communication with the pharmacist who will be providing care for their mutual clients. [IV]

 b. The physician and the pharmacist who will provide MMT client care agree upon suitable ways to share information with each other regarding their clients' progress in treatment and any adjustments needed to treatment plans. [IV]

3. Pharmacists in different treatment settings communicate and collaborate effectively about their mutual MMT clients during transitions in care, to increase client safety. [IV]

PHARMACY ENVIRONMENT AND CLIENT PERSPECTIVES

These recommendations address the first three questions posed by the panel at the beginning of the development process:

- What knowledge and skills and attitudes do pharmacists need to provide optimal MMT services safely to opioid-dependent clients?
- What is required in the pharmacy practice environment to ensure optimal MMT services?
- What can MMT clients expect from the care they receive from pharmacists and pharmacy practice sites?

The panel recommends that:

4. Pharmacy managers/owners offering MMT services ensure that the pharmacy has a suitable private area for respectful dosing and confidential discussion with clients. [III]

5. Pharmacy managers/owners ensure that all staff (professional and non-professional) employ the same respectful, professional approaches and attitudes toward MMT clients as they would use toward any other client of the pharmacy. [III]

6. The pharmacy have a treatment agreement with every client who is beginning methadone maintenance treatment at the pharmacy. [IV]

7. Pharmacy managers/owners inform relief pharmacists or new pharmacists that the practice site offers MMT services so that the pharmacists can ensure they are adequately prepared to offer this service. [IV]

8. Pharmacy managers ensure that there is a good system for communication among pharmacists within their practice environment regarding clients' treatment. [IV]

ACCESSIBILITY OF MMT PHARMACY SERVICES

These recommendations address the fourth question posed by the panel at the beginning of the development process:

- What is needed to ensure that MMT pharmacy services are available across Ontario?

The panel recommends that:

9. The Ontario College of Pharmacists, in conjunction with a professional pharmacy organization or CAMH, develop a mechanism for tracking pharmacies providing MMT services throughout the province, with the objective of identifying areas where there is little or no access to service. [IV]

10. Researchers survey pharmacists, particularly those in under-serviced regions, for their views and concerns about participating or not participating in MMT provision, with the goal of finding ways to encourage pharmacies throughout Ontario to provide MMT services and to support those currently providing MMT services. [III]

11. Researchers study the efficacy of offering incentives to pharmacists in remote or under-serviced areas to begin a methadone practice. [III]

12. Researchers work with the Ontario Pharmacy Council or a professional pharmacy organization to investigate fair and equitable payment models for MMT pharmacy services. [III]

13. The Local Health Integration Networks and addiction and mental health networks in under-serviced regions encourage and support initiatives to

increase MMT availability. Pharmacists in these areas can be invited to participate with other local health professionals, public health service providers and local hospitals to explore ways in which their communities could provide MMT dispensing and pharmacy services to people with opioid dependence. [IV]

14. Hospitals and other institutions (e.g., jails and prisons, long-term care facilities) ensure that they are able to meet the medication needs of persons maintained on methadone who are admitted to their facilities, and specifically that:

a. Pharmacists in these environments have the appropriate knowledge and skills to ensure safe provision of methadone services. [IV]

b. Pharmacists communicate and collaborate intraprofessionally during their mutual clients' transitions into or out of institutions to ensure they have safe and uninterrupted access to methadone treatment. [IV]

c. These institutions provide access, monitoring and pharmacy care services for their clients on methadone as they would for any other client. [IV]

PHARMACIST EDUCATION IN MMT

These recommendations address the first and fourth questions posed by the panel at the beginning of the development process:

- What knowledge and skills and attitudes do pharmacists need to provide optimal MMT services safely to opioid-dependent clients?
- What is needed to ensure that MMT pharmacy services are available across Ontario?

The panel recommends that:

15. Pharmacy managers/owners, hospital pharmacy directors and the Ontario College of Pharmacists support and encourage pharmacists providing methadone services to have education in and/or demonstrate knowledge and skills in core competency areas. These areas include:

a. Substance use disorders, including opioid dependence. [IV]

b. The varied models of substance abuse treatment, including harm reduction and its implications for pharmacy. [IV]

c. The impact of attitudes and stigma on client care. [III]

d. Methadone maintenance treatment clinical guidelines and their rationale, particularly with respect to practices to protect client safety, including:

- assessing initial and increased doses for appropriateness
- assessing methadone-dosing histories (for missed doses and irregularities in pattern of pickup) before dispensing a dose of methadone to a client
- ensuring the safe provision of "carries" (take-home doses) to clients
- dealing with intoxicated clients, including understanding the risks of polysubstance abuse. [IV]

16. All pharmacy students receive education on substance abuse, including opioid dependence, its treatment and practical intervention strategies, in their undergraduate curriculum. [IV]

17. Professional organizations, addiction and mental health agencies and pharmacists' employers promote the development of, and provide encouragement for all practising pharmacists to participate in, educational events on substance abuse and opioid dependence, including the growing problem of prescription opioid abuse. [III]

18. The Ontario College of Pharmacists revise the current requirements for pharmacies providing MMT services to mandate earlier training to promote safety. The designated manager and one pharmacist must complete the training within six months of starting to dispense methadone. [IV]

19. CAMH or another approved provider of methadone training develop a brief electronic document (e.g., one page) outlining the key safety features of providing MMT services that can be made available for immediate use by pharmacies initiating MMT services. [IV]

20. CAMH produce an electronic version of its most recent pharmacist's guide to methadone maintenance treatment that can be purchased online and downloaded immediately so that pharmacies initiating MMT services can access it without delay. [IV]

21. CAMH make the online component of its Opioid Dependence Treatment Course available immediately upon enrolment to pharmacists new to

providing MMT services, with the stipulation that these pharmacists attend the workshop component within six months of beginning the course. [IV]

22. CAMH or another approved provider of methadone training monitor and respond to waiting lists for training programs by, for example, offering the training more frequently or by exploring other delivery methods, such as webinars or video conferencing, to help meet the needs of pharmacists in remote areas. [IV]

23. The Ontario College of Pharmacists and providers of methadone training collaborate on ongoing training requirements based on needs identified during the College's pharmacy inspection process. [IV]

24. CAMH or another approved provider of methadone education deliver methadone training in a manner consistent with interprofessional education principles. [IV]

25. The Ontario College of Pharmacists and community colleges providing pharmacy technician training develop core competency requirements for regulated pharmacy technicians providing MMT services. [IV]

26. CAMH or another approved provider of methadone education undertake a needs assessment of pharmacists who have participated in the initial MMT training, and then use this information to develop an updated or advanced MMT course for pharmacists. [IV]

27. Professional pharmacy organizations, the Ontario College of Pharmacists, pharmacy managers/owners and hospital pharmacy directors encourage pharmacists to take courses on motivational interviewing, intervention strategies to use with difficult patients, and concurrent disorders, to enhance pharmacists' skills in dealing with opioid-dependent clients. [IV]

28. Drug information service providers ensure that staff is trained on and familiar with common issues in MMT treatment and have a mechanism to refer to experts when necessary. [IV]

29. Professional pharmacy organizations develop a mechanism in conjunction with the Ontario College of Pharmacists to ensure that pharmacists dispensing methadone are informed in a timely fashion of new educational resources available. [IV]

30. Professional pharmacy organizations, CAMH and funding agencies develop a mentorship program to link new methadone service providers with experienced providers. [IV]

31. Professional pharmacy organizations and CAMH promote the CAMH Addiction Clinical Consultation Service to pharmacists providing MMT services. [IV]

RESEARCH IN MMT PHARMACY PRACTICE

These recommendations address all four questions posed by the panel at the beginning of the development process:

- What knowledge and skills and attitudes do pharmacists need to provide optimal MMT services safely to opioid-dependent clients?
- What is required in the pharmacy practice environment to ensure optimal MMT services?
- What can MMT clients expect from the care they receive from pharmacists and pharmacy practice sites?
- What is needed to ensure that MMT pharmacy services are available across Ontario?

In addition to recommendations #10, 11 and 12, the panel recommends that:

32. Scientists in Ontario develop a research program to investigate all aspects of pharmacy practice in MMT, including:

a. the effectiveness of different models of care (including those with pharmacists in community pharmacies and in clinic settings)

b. the impact of pharmacist interventions on client outcomes

c. pharmacoeconomic implications

d. factors that could affect community pharmacy capacity to accommodate MMT clients

e. possible ways to increase access to methadone pharmacy services in remote areas. [IV]

33. Investigators study the impact of educational initiatives on patient outcomes. [IV]

Interprofessional collaboration and communication

Community pharmacists provide a significant point of contact as part of primary health care services and have regular (often daily) contact with the patient. Hence their role in the care of drug misusers is crucial and communication in both directions between pharmacists and other health care professionals should be encouraged.
                    —Shared Care Monitoring Group (2005, September)

Methadone maintenance treatment (MMT) involves shared care of the client by a team of many individuals. The MMT team consists of the client; the primary care team, including the prescribing physicians, the dispensing pharmacists, MMT program nurses and other program staff; case managers; and often community social service support workers. The client's optimal care and safety are the focus of each team member.

THE ROLE OF THE PHARMACIST

The panel recommends that:
1. MMT programs and methadone prescribers recognize the role of pharmacists in collaborative care and this role's impact on their mutual clients' treatment. Specifically, the College of Physicians and Surgeons of Ontario should emphasize in its *Methadone Maintenance Guidelines* the importance of collaboration and regular communication with the pharmacist and their impact on patient care and safety. [IV]

The pharmacist is a member of the health care team in primary care and the most accessible member of the team to clients. Pharmacist-specific roles include dispensing methadone, observing and assessing clients, supervising methadone ingestion and tracking adherence. Other components of the pharmacist's role are educating clients about methadone, including its potential adverse and toxic effects, how and why doses are increased slowly, and the importance of not missing doses, especially during the early stages of treatment. The pharmacist also orients clients to the routine in the pharmacy and has a treatment agreement with each MMT client outlining each party's expectations. The pharmacist develops a relationship with his or her MMT clients, seeing the clients daily in the first few months of treatment, which is more frequently than the clients see the physician, program staff or case manager. These brief encounters, especially at the start of treatment, provide important opportunities for motivating clients, promoting health and providing support or intervention when needed (New Brunswick Addiction Services, 2005). These daily encounters also allow the pharmacist to develop an overall impression of how the client is progressing in treatment.

> The pharmacist's brief daily encounters with clients provide opportunities, particularly at the start of MMT, to motivate clients, promote health, provide support and intervene when needed. These opportunities are especially important when the client is starting treatment.

CHALLENGES IN SHARED CARE

The pharmacist has valuable contributions to make to the MMT client's care but pharmacists working in community pharmacies face challenges related to collaborative practice. Communication with other members of the health care team can be a significant challenge. Because the pharmacist often works at a different location, he or she does not have easy proximity to other team members for consultation. These team members, particularly the prescribing physicians, may be difficult to reach. As well, pharmacists work with different teams for each client, and each team may have several different members. Furthermore, the community pharmacist's contributions to clients' treatment may be underestimated by the prescribing physician or treatment program staff. MMT programs and methadone prescribers need to understand the roles of community pharmacists and their contribution to their mutual clients' treatment. Pharmacists should, in the context of their regular communication with other team member colleagues, educate prescribers and other health care providers about the knowledge, skills and expertise that pharmacists have that can complement their treatment of MMT clients, with the goal of optimal outcomes for each individual client.

IMPACT OF SHARED CARE

Interprofessional collaboration and a multidisciplinary approach to mental health care, including MMT services, have the potential to improve the health outcomes of clients. In shared care, health professionals from different professions work with clients in planned, interdependent collaboration (Curnan et al., 2006; HealthForceOntario, 2007). The team-based approach is designed to ensure that clients receive co-ordinated, quality care.

The importance of establishing interprofessional communication and collaboration is consistently supported in methadone treatment clinical practice guidelines (Health Canada, 2002).

For example, the New Brunswick Addiction Services' *Methadone Maintenance Treatment Guidelines* (2005) state that direct collaboration between and among MMT team members and clients helps achieve the treatment goals of reducing harms of drug use, treating comorbidity and helping clients achieve higher levels of psychosocial function. The New Brunswick *Guidelines* and other guidelines from British Columbia (College of Pharmacists of British Columbia, 2007) also recommend that all team members, including pharmacists, demonstrate a willingness to participate fully with each other in order to contribute to their clients' success.

In Glasgow in the United Kingdom, the methadone program name was changed to the "Shared Care Programme" to indicate that this treatment is a joint venture between medical, social and pharmaceutical services (Glasgow City Council, 2008).

The panel recommends that:

2. Prescribing physicians and MMT programs establish and then maintain communication with community pharmacists regarding client treatment plans and progress. [IV] In particular, the panel recommends that:

> **a. At the outset of MMT, the prescribing physician initiate contact and communication with the pharmacist who will be providing care for their mutual clients. [IV]**
>
> **b. The physician and the pharmacist who will provide MMT client care agree upon suitable ways to share information with each other regarding their clients' progress in treatment and any adjustments needed to treatment plans. [IV]**

The importance of establishing an interprofessional working relationship between the prescribing physician and the pharmacist at the initiation of the client's treatment is supported by the Collège des médecins du Québec & Ordre des pharmaciens du Québec (2000) and by the College of Pharmacists of B.C. (2007). Their guidelines recommend that at the start of treatment the prescribing physician contact the pharmacist of the client's choice who will be providing methadone services.

Initial contact between physician and pharmacist should include discussion about the client's needs (for example, other health issues, polysubstance use, concurrent disorders) and whether the pharmacist can accommodate the client's treatment in his or her pharmacy practice. It is also the opportunity for the community pharmacist to establish a solid working relationship with the prescriber. This first contact allows communication regarding further contact as the need arises.

For shared care to work well, team members need to develop suitable ways of sharing information during assessment and treatment planning and for communicating clinical feedback that may necessitate adjustments in treatment over time. Where a pharmacy has several pharmacists providing MMT, one pharmacist could be designated to be the main contact for a particular client except in the case of an urgent issue.

Keene et al. (2004) describe the positive effect shared care can have on team members' satisfaction in their working relationships, as well as its beneficial impact on client treatment outcomes. For example, the authors describe a program delivering shared care and treatment to opioid-dependent clients in Berkshire, England, who were prescribed methadone. The program involved collaboration among prescribing physicians, pharmacists, drug agency workers and patients. In this survey, the professionals experienced unanimity in their satisfaction working with opioid-dependent clients and attributed this satisfaction to feeling more secure treating clients on methadone because they had "backup" from their colleagues and shared the responsibility for the clients' care. After treatment started, clients visited the physicians every two weeks and had contact with the pharmacists daily for supervised methadone dosing. The pharmacists involved in this shared care program reported satisfaction in being able to see their clients achieve stability and improve their lifestyles.

In Keene et al. (2004), the pharmacists surveyed felt that shared care had improved their working relationships but still identified a pressing need to further improve communications between professionals and to work out better systems for transferring information.

Physicians need to access clinical information acquired by community pharmacists about their clients to make important treatment decisions, for example, regarding methadone doses, take-home status and continuity of care. For example, a physician unaware that a client missed methadone every other day of the week may increase a dose because the client complains of withdrawal.

> Physicians need to access clinical information acquired by community pharmacists about their clients to make important treatment decisions. Good communication between the prescribing physician and the community pharmacist benefits patient care.

In Li's survey of 16 pharmacists in Toronto (1996), maintaining good communication with physicians was perceived as a must for monitoring clients' progress in treatment. The majority of the pharmacists (78 per cent) responded that they would confirm the prescription with the prescriber.

The other most common reasons for contact with the prescriber were to report missed doses, to advise about suspected substance abuse and to discuss possible drug interactions. In this survey, pharmacists reported that where there was poor communication, client problems arose. Sometimes miscommunication occurred because physicians had expectations of the pharmacist (for example, that the pharmacist would be involved in urine drug screening) that they had not clarified either verbally or in writing. A communication from the prescriber at the start of treatment would be a time for agreement between the pharmacist and prescriber regarding management of their mutual client.

Although pharmacists are an important part of the primary care team, many pharmacists anecdotally report that they often don't feel that they are part of the team, and that most information sharing is one-way, to the prescriber. Pharmacists have little contact with the prescriber or MMT clinic unless there are problems. Lack of feedback from prescribers and programs and difficulty accessing physicians when problems develop enforce this impression held by many pharmacists.

Physicians and programs that provide feedback to pharmacists about how shared client information affected client care strengthen the foundation of collaboration and facilitate further communication. When this communication occurs, pharmacists feel more positive and involved in their client's treatment, and consequently feel encouraged to share more useful information. When pharmacists don't receive a response, they may be wary of contacting the prescriber when it is essential (Bond, 2000).

MMT programs can invite the pharmacist to participate in patient case conferences and educational activities. Although it may not be practical for some in community practice to attend regular meetings, MMT programs' efforts to include pharmacists could significantly benefit client care.

The panel recommends that:
3. Pharmacists in different treatment settings communicate and collaborate effectively about their mutual MMT clients during transitions in care, to increase client safety. [IV]

During transition in a client's care, such as when a client is changing community pharmacies or admitted or discharged from a hospital or jail, there should be intraprofessional collaboration between the different pharmacy sites. Pharmacists must be vigilant about communication with other pharmacists at each and every transition in MMT care and they must clearly document the communication in the patient record.

Serious medication errors may result when this communication does not occur, with clinical consequences for the client. Without this communication, there is a risk that the client could receive a double dose of methadone, or too high an individual dose after a loss of tolerance from a period of missed doses. The clinical effects on the client can range from intoxication and sedation to overdose and death. For example, in one such case in Ontario known to the panel, there was no communication between a new pharmacy taking over a client's MMT care and the previous dispensing pharmacy. Unfortunately, this client had not received methadone for five days at the previous pharmacy and was given the usual prescribed dose, which led to a methadone overdose, and the client sustained serious neurological damage. Communication between pharmacists can reduce the risk of harm to the MMT client during transitions in care.

Pharmacy environment and client perspectives

A non-judgemental and non-stigmatising attitude towards this area of health care is an essential starting point for quality care.
—*Sheridan and Strang (2003, p. 1)*

The pharmacy environment includes everything from the location of the pharmacy and the physical layout of the premises to the attitudes and services provided. All of these factors may influence a client's decision to attend a particular pharmacy and may have an impact on his or her satisfaction with treatment. The panel recognizes that in some communities, especially non-urban or remote areas of Ontario, there may be few options or even only one. Studies have found that MMT clients choose a pharmacy for the same reasons as other consumers, for example, because the pharmacy's location is convenient, close to work, school or home (Anstice et al., 2009; Luger et al., 2000; Matheson, 2003). These studies also identified longer operating hours, which allow clients to carry on with activities of daily living such as parenting or working, to be an important factor. However, in other respects MMT clients' needs are unique. Because they take their medication daily in the pharmacy under observation, they have special requirements beyond the normal courtesy any pharmacy customer might expect, and they desire treatment that is discreet, quick and non-judgmental (Matheson, 2003).

PRIVACY

FROM THE CLIENT CONSULTATION INTERVIEWS

CLIENTS TALK ABOUT PRIVACY

"We need more privacy when drinking meds or talking about an issue."

"There should be a lot more privacy, to fully separate areas for discussion and pickup. I don't want everybody to hear."

"They have a side room but they don't use it. It doesn't bother me but for some people, it might bother them."

The panel recommends that:
4. Pharmacy managers/owners offering MMT services ensure that the pharmacy has a suitable private area for respectful dosing and confidential discussion with clients. [III]

Pharmacies should be a safe place for methadone clients, other patients of the pharmacy and pharmacy staff. In this context "safety" means an environment in which people can feel secure not only physically but also free from social or emotional threats such as loss of privacy or stigma-tization. For MMT clients, a private space in which to take their dose of methadone or to consult the pharmacist is an important issue. Indeed, privacy and confidentiality are important for every patient, and many pharmacies are responding by creating a private area where clients may consult with the pharmacist about treatment or services in confidence.

Some MMT clients feel strongly about the need for privacy in the pharmacy, while others may be comfortable as long as they are treated with respect and discretion by the pharmacist. In a qualitative study, Anstice et al. (2009) interviewed MMT clients from four methadone programs in Ontario. Their findings confirmed that clients valued discreet service and privacy in the pharmacy for their observed doses.

In Luger et al.'s survey of methadone clients in London, England (2000), 60 per cent of the respondents said they did not feel comfortable drinking methadone in the pharmacy because they felt embarrassed and concerned that their conversations with the pharmacist could be overhead by other customers and staff. In response, some pharmacists asked clients to come at a time when the pharmacy was likely to be less busy. Some offered dispensing at a quiet corner of the store. The ability of many pharmacies to respond to this concern was limited because their premises did not offer a private area.

Lea et al. (2008) surveyed 508 clients in New South Wales, Australia, regarding their satisfaction with opioid treatment services provided by their pharmacy. Clients reported a high level of service in many areas, giving their pharmacies a mean rating above eight out of 10 on a number of aspects, with 10 indicating best service. These aspects included:
- safety
- staff quality
- confidentiality
- fair and consistent service
- opening and closing hours.

However, clients reported less satisfaction with the privacy available to them during supervised dosing. In spite of the clients' overall positive scoring of their pharmacies' services, 25 per cent felt that they were not treated the same as other customers and 35 per cent reported having to wait longer than other customers and sometimes being made to wait while others were served first.

Pharmacists could discuss clients' preferences with them so as to increase the clients' comfort and to avoid embarrassment or misunderstandings. If no private area exists, pharmacists can discuss with the client his or her feelings about taking the dose in view of others. If clients are not comfortable taking the dose in view of others, pharmacists and clients may discuss the client arranging to come during a time of day when the pharmacy is quiet, rather than at peak hours; others may arrange that the client wait until other customers are out of view before taking the dose. For some clients there may be additional reasons to choose a pharmacy where they have less likelihood of seeing other MMT clients with whom they may have used drugs in the past. In the study by Anstice et al. (2009) of MMT clients in Ontario, some clients preferred to avoid dispensing sites where they could meet other MMT clients and the triggers to use drugs that resulted from being with others who were still using or dealing in drugs.

ATTITUDES AND BEHAVIOURS

Most clients want to be treated like any other patient of the pharmacy. Neale (1998) interviewed 124 clients in Scotland about their thoughts on pharmacy providers. The way that pharmacy staff behaved toward the client was considered an important part of the service delivered; in this study, female clients more frequently identified the importance of this behaviour. A good pharmacy service was described as one in which the clients felt they were treated like any other customer, where the service was friendly, discreet and confidential. In general, clients disliked intrusive questions. Clients valued ordinary interaction such as chatting about day-to-day issues and developing a personal rapport with the pharmacist and pharmacy staff. Clients in this survey preferred community pharmacies over centralized clinics. Although these clients considered their prescribers more important than the pharmacists in their treatment, they rated the physicians as less helpful.

FROM THE CLIENT CONSULTATION INTERVIEWS

CLIENTS TALK ABOUT PHARMACY EXPERIENCES

"Be more understanding about people on methadone. [At the pharmacy] they put other customers first. Sometimes I've waited all day to have my methadone prescription filled. By 3:00 p.m. I'm feeling rough . . . when I dropped it off at 9:00 a.m."

"Some staff aren't very nice. You get the feeling that they say 'Here comes another junkie.' You can feel when someone has an attitude."

"I've overheard staff talking about other clients and laughing at them. It was very inappropriate."

"I would be at the front of the line at the pharmacy and then often people would come after me and get served first. I told them I didn't like it and we worked it out. It's been better for the last month."

"The pharmacy staff was very helpful when I started out. They were very encouraging. I didn't feel well at first but they helped me hang in there."

"They are really friendly; they phone the doctor for me about my other medication."

"Being in line for pharmacy isn't good. People fight physically, deal drugs, talk about drugs. You see bad things when you are trying to get sober. It's easy for me to get drugs here. The scene here can be very intense. It's not a safe place, especially for children. Mothers bring children here."

Pharmacies have other patients (not on MMT) who also have treatment needs that should not be affected by their pharmacy dispensing methadone. Lawrie et al. (2004) interviewed 80 customers (of 10 stores providing MMT services) in Glasgow to explore their attitudes about using a pharmacy that offers MMT services. One of the findings was that most were sympathetic toward drug misusers and had a fairly positive attitude toward methadone maintenance treatment. Although much of the customers' knowledge about MMT was acquired from media reports and many of the customers did not have a clear understanding of why people were on MMT, most recognized that MMT clients should have some privacy in the pharmacy for taking their doses. This survey did not find that customers were deterred by a pharmacy's dispensing methadone to MMT clients; in fact, some of the customers were not even aware that their pharmacy offered MMT services.

The panel recommends that:
5. Pharmacy managers/owners ensure that all staff (professional and non-professional) employ the same respectful, professional approaches and attitudes toward MMT clients as they would use toward any other client of the pharmacy. [III]

Pharmacy staff should treat all clients of the pharmacy in a positive, respectful, non-judgmental and professional manner. The manner in which a pharmacist interacts with an MMT client often affects the way the client deals with the pharmacist and staff (Matheson, Bond & Hickey, 1999).

GIVE RESPECT TO GET RESPECT

When interactions are positive and professional and clients receive the same respectful treatment as other customers, pharmacists can develop a rapport with their MMT clients.

When interactions are positive and professional, pharmacists can develop a rapport with their MMT clients (Matheson, 2003). The effect of the pharmacist and staff of the pharmacy on the MMT client can be considerable. Many clients already feel stigmatized by society and in some encounters with other health care providers involved in their treatment. Because the first visit to the pharmacy in MMT involves a lengthy period of time for establishing identification, completing the pharmacist-client agreement, discussing routines and so on, many clients may be frustrated with the time it takes to get their methadone dose. When pharmacists acknowledge this issue and proceed in a non-judgmental, friendly manner, they convey respect for the client (Matheson, 2003).

In surveys about pharmacists' attitudes and practices, there was an association between positive attitude scores and professional practice activities such as preparing methadone doses in advance and treating MMT clients the same as other customers. Pharmacists who had taken training in opioid-dependence treatment had higher attitude scores than those who had not (Matheson, Bond & Mollison, 1999; Matheson et al., 2002; Sheridan & Barber, 1997; Sheridan et al., 2007).

FROM THE CLIENT CONSULTATION INTERVIEWS

CLIENTS REPORT ON PHARMACY CARE EXPERIENCES

- 80% reported that the lack of privacy (taking their medication or talking to the pharmacist in a public rather than private space) was the most challenging issue for them at pharmacies.
- 17% had access to a private area in the pharmacy for discussion with the pharmacist.
- 22% had access to a private area for taking their methadone dose.
- 58% had a written agreement with their pharmacist.
- 90% reported that a caring attitude and courteous, non-judgmental staff were the most positive aspects of dealing with the pharmacies where they drank their methadone.
- Nearly 30% reported rude or judgmental staff during pharmacy service.
- 26% had an educational session with the pharmacist before treatment began.

The panel recommends that:
6. The pharmacy have a treatment agreement with every client who is beginning methadone maintenance treatment at the pharmacy. [IV]

To ensure safety of clients and pharmacy staff, outlining each party's expectations of behaviour in the pharmacy is an important component of the treatment agreement. When done early in treatment, it encourages mutual respect between clients and staff and provides agreed boundaries. Pharmacists should spend time verbally reviewing the written agreement and clarifying any issues with the client. When the pharmacist receives advance notice from the prescriber/MMT team about a new client starting treatment at the pharmacy, he or she can set aside appropriate time for this review with the client.

The agreement can outline what the client can expect from the pharmacy and what the pharmacy can expect from the client. It can outline appropriate behaviour in the pharmacy so that the pharmacy is a safe place for the client, other clients and staff. To avoid the development of problematic behaviours, the treatment agreement can provide information such as, but not limited to, what the client can expect if doses are missed or if the client arrives at the pharmacy intoxicated. The treatment agreement could also address issues of loitering or drug dealing in the vicinity of the pharmacy.

The panel recommends that:
7. Pharmacy managers/owners inform relief pharmacists or new pharmacists that the practice site offers MMT services so that the pharmacists can ensure they are adequately prepared to offer this service. [IV]

Pharmacy managers should as much as possible hire new or relief staff that have taken the appropriate training (Sutcliffe, 2009). The appropriate MMT reference materials and written pharmacy store policies should be readily available to new or relief pharmacists starting at the pharmacy.

The panel recommends that:
8. Pharmacy managers ensure that there is a good system for communication among pharmacists within their practice environment regarding clients' treatment. [IV]

It should be clear to a pharmacist starting a shift at the pharmacy if there are any outstanding issues or clinical concerns regarding a client's methadone treatment. For example, some pharmacies use a communication book to highlight unresolved concerns and to prepare pharmacists coming on to a shift.

Accessibility of MMT pharmacy services

THE INTERNATIONAL PERSPECTIVE

The involvement of pharmacists in providing opioid maintenance treatment (methadone and buprenorphine) has been rapidly expanding over the last decade in many countries. In Ireland, Australia, New Zealand, the United Kingdom and other European countries (e.g., Switzerland, Germany, Spain and Portugal) there is an extensive push for pharmacists' involvement (Berbatis et al., 2003; Gastelurrutia et al., 2005; Neilson, 2007; Samitca et al., 2007).

In Scotland, Matheson et al. conducted several surveys at five-year intervals of all pharmacies in the country (Matheson, Bond & Hickey, 1999; Matheson, Bond & Mollison, 1999; Matheson et al., 2002; Matheson et al., 2007) and found that the proportion of pharmacies providing MMT service increased from 53 per cent to 79 per cent over 10 years. By the midpoint of the study the mean number of clients per pharmacy had increased from 7 to 20 (Matheson, Bond & Hickey, 1999; Matheson et al., 2002). Mackie et al. (2004) compared pharmacy involvement in Dublin and Glasgow. They found that 80 per cent of pharmacies in Dublin provided MMT services, compared to 38 per cent of pharmacies in Glasgow. In a survey of all pharmacies (2,473) in England, Sheridan et al. (2007)

found an increase in the proportion of pharmacies providing opioid substitution therapy (mostly methadone), from 51 per cent in 1995 to 63 per cent in 2005. The average number of clients per pharmacy increased from 5.9 to 9.2 over this time period.

Lawrinson et al. (2008) reported that in 2005 88 per cent of opioid substitution treatment clients in South Australia received their medication through pharmacies, three per cent received their medication from public clinics and the rest received their medication through prison pharmacies. Almost half of all pharmacies in this region were providing opioid substitution therapy services. The mean number of patients per pharmacy was seven in metropolitan areas and four in rural areas. In Victoria, Australia, 95 per cent of all opioid substitution pharmacotherapy is provided by community pharmacies (Nielson, 2007).

In contrast, in the United States there is little involvement of pharmacies in providing methadone for opioid dependence, due to jurisprudence. Methadone is primarily provided through specialized clinics. There are some models of community pharmacy involvement in several small pilots around the country (in New Mexico; Lancaster County, Pennsylvania; New York City; Seattle, Washington) in which pharmacists have taken training and collaborate with local physicians to provide service to stabilized methadone patients (Drucker et al., 2007; Tuchman, 2008; Tuchman et al., 2003).

AVAILABILITY IN ONTARIO

In Ontario, as of June 2009, 549 of 3,253 pharmacies (17 per cent) provided MMT services (personal communication, OCP, June 29, 2009). The total number of clients maintained on methadone, as of early July 2009, was 23,852, and there were 276 prescribers (personal communication, CPSO, July 2, 2009). It is unclear how many clients are receiving their methadone from community pharmacies and how many through clinics.

The panel recommends that:

9. The Ontario College of Pharmacists, in conjunction with a professional pharmacy organization or CAMH, develop a mechanism for tracking pharmacies providing MMT services throughout the province, with the objective of identifying areas where there is little or no access to service. [IV]

Information regarding the locations of pharmacies dispensing methadone should be available for research, education and training purposes. Procedures for ensuring the confidentiality of this information can be included in the system developed. Findings from this research will help in identifying needs for expanding availability through pharmacies in Ontario. The Ontario College of Pharmacists could involve other organizations, for example, CAMH or the Ontario Pharmacists' Association, in the development and maintenance of this system.

Such data is currently available in British Columbia. The College of Pharmacists of British Columbia reports that 52 per cent of pharmacies in the province dispense methadone. Information about regional distribution is also available: 56 per cent of pharmacies in the Lower Mainland dispense methadone for maintenance treatment, and 20 per cent dispense on Vancouver Island (Budd & McClelland, 2006). The panel recognizes that British Columbia is less populous than Ontario and has far fewer pharmacies.

In British Columbia, the College of Pharmacists also maintains a website with a referral list of pharmacies that have asked to have their contact information made available. The list gives the address, phone number and hours of operation for each of these pharmacies. This information helps clients find a pharmacy that is convenient and appropriate for their health care needs. Some pharmacies providing MMT have decided not to have their name posted on the College website.

The panel recommends that:

10. Researchers survey pharmacists, particularly those in under-serviced regions, for their views and concerns about participating or not participating in MMT provision, with the goal of finding ways to encourage

pharmacies throughout Ontario to provide MMT services and to support those currently providing MMT services. [III]

The concerns and views of pharmacists working in areas where there is limited or no access to MMT services need to be considered in any planning by service advocates. Researching and then addressing these issues will help to remove barriers to more widespread provision of methadone for opioid-dependent clients throughout the province and enable the involvement of pharmacists in MMT treatment. Current resources, such as the MethadoneSavesLives.ca website, offer information, education and support to pharmacists in Ontario considering the provision of methadone services. As survey results become available, these resources could be modified to include those concerns and views of pharmacists not currently addressed.

It is important to remember that professional pharmacy organizations and the OCP can support pharmacies already providing MMT and encourage their continued provision of this service by surveying them about and then by addressing their concerns, problems and needs. For example, learning about pharmacists' concerns and needs alerts education providers to address these areas, or suggests to policy-makers amendments that could be made to MMT policies or guidelines.

Mackie et al. (2004) and Roberts et al. (2007), in their surveys of pharmacists in Glasgow and Dublin, found that the most frequent reasons pharmacists gave for not providing service were:
- business reasons, including risks to staff and property
- concern that other customers might object
- lack of suitable area for dosing
- they were too busy to provide an efficient service
- the company or owner didn't want to.

Mackie et al. also surveyed non-providers, asking what would encourage them to provide MMT service in the future. Those responding said that they would consider providing this service in the future if:
- there was an increased demand for such a service
- the service was confined to the local area only

- there was good co-operation between local general practitioners and local pharmacists
- there was increased pharmacy security
- there was a controlled, established scheme of prescribing guidelines.

These findings are similar to those of Sheridan et al. in 2007.

One of the concerns common among non-providers was that providing service might affect care they provided for other customers of the pharmacy. However, interestingly, Lawrie et al. (2004) conducted a survey of the views of other customers and found that they were generally supportive of their community pharmacies providing this service as long as MMT clients were given privacy for dosing.

The panel recommends that:
11. Researchers study the efficacy of offering incentives to pharmacists in remote or under-serviced areas to begin a methadone practice. [III]

International research has identified security concerns such as theft and risk to staff and property as important for pharmacists considering methadone dispensing. Roberts et al. (2007) in Glasgow described ways to potentially address these concerns, such as increased funding for pharmacies to install panic buttons or a closed-circuit television system. This study also recommended a program that would provide special funding for renovation of pharmacies in certain regions so that they could create a private area suitable for dispensing methadone.

Sheridan et al. (2007), having surveyed activities and attitudes of pharmacists across England, attributed the increase in pharmacy involvement in MMT to increased government funding for opioid substitution, including adequate compensation for pharmacies providing MMT services and financial support for pharmacist MMT training.

The panel recommends that:
12. Researchers work with the Ontario Pharmacy Council or a professional pharmacy organization to investigate fair and equitable payment models for MMT pharmacy services. [III]

This recommendation is consistent with the Ontario Ministry of Health and Long-Term Care's *Methadone Task Force Report* recommendation that the Ontario Pharmacy Council determine, and advise the ministry on, the most appropriate funding model to encourage pharmacists to dispense MMT (Hart, 2007).

Any methadone payment model should recognize the value of methadone services provided by pharmacists and the considerable workload involved in this service (e.g., supervising dosing daily, checking for missed doses, assessing for intoxication, communication with the prescribing physician, monitoring and brief counselling of clients and managing the critical safety issues). The compensation should be fair payment for the unique elements involved in providing methadone services.

When pharmacists are appropriately reimbursed for MMT services, they are more likely to consider offering it. Sheridan et al. (2007) attributed some of the increase in pharmacist MMT service provision in England between 1995 and 2005 to an increase in remuneration. Inadequate compensation for pharmacists' involvement has been described as a major barrier to recruiting pharmacies to provide MMT services in Australia (Peterson, 1999).

Some elements of models used in other provinces can be explored when considering the question of appropriate compensation for methadone dispensing services in Ontario. For example, since 2001 in British Columbia, PharmaCare has included a special interaction fee for the unusual elements involved in supervising methadone dosing. Further, in British Columbia there is a refusal-to-dispense program that permits pharmacists to claim a dispensing fee under certain circumstances if the pharmacist judges that it is in the best interest of the patient that the prescription not be dispensed (FCH, 2007).

Quebec has a general payment model for cognitive services provided by a pharmacist. Using this mechanism, pharmacists are reimbursed for providing a pharmaceutical opinion. This payment involves the pharmacist providing documentation of appropriate communication with the physician—that is, a notice or a letter to the physician with the aim of modifying the prescribed treatment. In Quebec, as in British Columbia, pharmacists receive payment for refusal to dispense (Kroger et al., 2000).

The panel recommends that:

13. The Local Health Integration Networks and addiction and mental health networks in under-serviced regions encourage and support initiatives to increase M M T availability. Pharmacists in these areas can be invited to participate with other local health professionals, public health service providers and local hospitals to explore ways in which their communities could provide M M T dispensing and pharmacy services to people with opioid dependence. [IV]

Pharmacists in community or hospital practice may have ideas for local solutions to under-servicing. These solutions may include collaborations among health care providers in the community to offer suitable service coverage or to discuss alternative service provision models, such as integration into hospital services. Merrill et al. (2005) describes hospital pharmacists working collaboratively with general practitioners in a general internal medicine clinic of a public hospital in the United States to provide care for stabilized methadone clients.

THE ROLE OF HOSPITALS AND INSTITUTIONS

In addition to exploring alternative service models with hospitals and other service providers in under-serviced areas, hospitals and other institutions need to ensure accessibility to methadone services for their clients who are in methadone maintenance treatment.

The panel recommends that:

14. Hospitals and other institutions (e.g., jails and prisons, long-term care facilities) ensure that they are able to meet the medication needs of persons maintained on methadone who are admitted to their facilities, and specifically that:

> **a. Pharmacists in these environments have the appropriate knowledge and skills to ensure safe provision of methadone services. [IV]**

b. Pharmacists communicate and collaborate intraprofessionally during their mutual clients' transitions into or out of institutions to ensure they have safe and uninterrupted access to methadone treatment. [IV]

c. These institutions provide access, monitoring and pharmacy care services for their clients on methadone as they would for any other client. [IV]

Hospitals and other institutions should have a policy on MMT in place to ensure continuity of treatment for methadone clients while they are under their care or within their walls. When no policy exists, the institution's pharmacist can play a role in the formulation and establishment of such a policy. Pharmacies within these institutions or pharmacists having contracts with these institutions should assist in formulating this policy when none is yet in place.

Pharmacists should also contribute to the education of staff at local institutions. When at least one pharmacist working at a site is trained, this pharmacist can be a resource for the rest of the pharmacy staff.

FROM THE CLIENT CONSULTATION INTERVIEWS

A CLIENT TALKS ABOUT METHADONE AND JAIL

"You can miss your drink for a few days when you're discharged from jail. It's not organized well. You don't get your drink the day you are released. If you go to court that day, you go without your drink. It's messed up. It's the jail's problem."

Medication reconciliation during transitions in care is an important patient safety issue (Canadian Patient Safety Institute, 2008), and this is particularly true for clients taking methadone. Pharmacists can assist with continuity of care and temporary exemption issues for the physician. For clients covered under the Ontario Drug Benefit (ODB) program, a list of medications dispensed is available in hospital settings to facilitate the medication reconciliation process. However, since methadone for MMT is prepared as an extemporaneous product in most pharmacies, there is inconsistency in how the product details appear in the ODB profiler listing. For example, panel members know of a near miss incident, where, upon a methadone client's admission to hospital, an entry of "100" was interpreted as the dose, and an order for methadone 100 mg was written. In accordance with the routine process the institution used when patients on methadone were admitted, it directly contacted the client's outside pharmacy prior to dose administration. The client's pharmacy clarified that the client's dose was actually much lower but had been dispensed in a 100 mL diluted solution. This example illustrates why hospitals and other facilities must have an established process in place to ensure methadone doses are confirmed directly with the client's last service provider.

Hospitals, long-term care facilities and other institutions should have established processes in place that are known to all clinical staff to facilitate the safe care of MMT clients. A clear process may help to reduce the anxiety staff have when uncertain about the best practices for the care of a client on methadone. Appropriate resources, including the CPSO's *Methadone Maintenance Treatment Guidelines* (2005) and CAMH's *Methadone Maintenance: A Pharmacist's Guide to Treatment* (Isaac et al., 2004), should be available for reference and consultation. Pharmacists working in these settings must be knowledgeable about methadone and demonstrate the core competencies required for safe methadone service provision (as outlined in the next section).

Pharmacist education in MMT

Pharmacists have the unique knowledge, skills and responsibilities for assuming an important role in substance abuse prevention education and assistance . . . Pharmacists, as health care providers, should be actively involved in reducing the negative effects that substance abuse has on society, health systems and the pharmacy profession.
—American Society of Health-System Pharmacists (2003)

COMPETENCY FRAMEWORK

Unless they have taken special training, most pharmacists are unaware of the clinical and practice issues surrounding methadone and their impact on client safety because they have had little or no exposure to them during their undergraduate pharmacy education.

The role of the pharmacist in MMT is unusual and there is no similar model in other therapeutic areas. Daily interactions with clients, along with direct clinical assessments, supervised dose administration and close monitoring do not usually occur in other types of pharmacy care. Pharmacists require a set of key competencies to ensure client safety in methadone maintenance treatment.

The panel recommends that:
15. Pharmacy managers/owners, hospital pharmacy directors and the Ontario College of Pharmacists support and encourage pharmacists providing methadone services to have education in and/or demonstrate knowledge and skills in core competency areas. These areas include:

a. Substance use disorders, including opioid dependence. [IV]
b. The varied models of substance abuse treatment, including harm reduction and its implications for pharmacy. [IV]
c. The impact of attitudes and stigma on client care. [III]
d. Methadone maintenance treatment clinical guidelines and their rationale, particularly with respect to practices to protect client safety, including:
- **assessing initial and increased doses for appropriateness**
- **assessing methadone-dosing histories (for missed doses and irregularities in pattern of pickup) before dispensing a dose of methadone to a client**
- **ensuring the safe provision of "carries" (take-home doses) to clients**
- **dealing with intoxicated clients, including understanding the risks of polysubstance abuse. [IV]**

Pharmacists need to understand substance use disorders, particularly addiction, and to understand the difference between "use" and "use disorders." Pharmacists need to be able to identify individuals with substance use disorders and to help motivate them to seek change and treatment. As one of the most accessible health care professionals, the pharmacist can play an important role and refer patients to appropriate services and substance use treatment programs. Many MMT clients have concurrent substance use disorders with substances such as alcohol, benzodiazepines or cocaine. Pharmacists should understand the risks associated with polysubstance use and the risk of toxicity.

Although pharmacists may already be involved in harm reduction, for example, by providing sterile needles and syringes to people who use injection drugs, further involvement could include offering advice to people with substance use problems about health issues and how to minimize health risks. A random survey of 2,017 Canadian pharmacists by Myers et al. (1998) found that while more than 88 per cent of pharmacists were comfortable with the harm reduction role in providing needles and syringes, this comfort did not extend to providing methadone services. This may be due to a misunderstanding of the benefits of methadone maintenance treatment and its role as a harm reduction approach. Educational initiatives need to address such misunderstandings and other negative attitudes or misperceptions that may be held by pharmacists.

Pharmacists must have a good understanding of the critical safety issues associated with methadone. Methadone has a unique pharmacological profile that makes it useful in the treatment of opioid dependence; however, it is different from other opioids and the implications of its long half-life can lead to risks of accumulation contributing to methadone overdose and deaths.

The initiation phase of methadone treatment can be a time of high risk for toxicity and pharmacists' understanding of dosing recommendations is critical at this stage. Pharmacists need to exercise particular vigilance in monitoring client dosing for appropriateness. For example, where clients have missed several doses (defined as three or more), or fewer (one or two) during periods of methadone dose escalation, pharmacists must understand the concept of loss of tolerance and risks to clients if the usual regular methadone dose is administered (CPSO, 2005).

Pharmacists also have to understand the safety issues associated with "carries." Having a written carry agreement with the client is one way to help the client understand these issues as well. Pharmacists should be aware of some of the signs that indicate a formerly stable client on a high level of carries is relapsing to instability (e.g., missing observed dosing days, lost carries) (CPSO, 2005).

Pharmacists in Ontario need to be familiar with the CPSO's most recent *Methadone Maintenance Guidelines* (2005), the OCP's *Policy for Dispensing Methadone* (2006), and CAMH's *Methadone Maintenance: A Pharmacist's Guide to Treatment* (Isaac et al., 2004).

Understanding the risks of polysubstance use and knowing how to deal with intoxicated clients are particularly important core competency areas for pharmacists, with significant safety implications. The pharmacist should have an understanding of the impact that polysubstance use (for example, use of benzodiazepines, alcohol and cocaine) can have on the client taking MMT. Through dialogue and checking for signs of excessive dosing or substance use such as sedation, slurring of speech, smelling of alcohol and unsteady gait, the pharmacist should be able to assess if a client is intoxicated before dosing.

Recommendations from the coroner have highlighted the need for assessing clients for intoxication because deaths have occurred through combination of methadone and other drugs, including alcohol (OCP, 2008).

In an Australian survey (Peterson et al., 2007), pharmacists identified the risk of overdose associated with methadone alone and in combination with other psychoactive drugs as the greatest problematic issue for pharmacists in deciding to provide a methadone service.

In a survey of 148 pharmacists in Australia (Koutroulis et al., 2000), when asked about how they would respond to clients who presented intoxicated for their methadone dose, 44 per cent said they would withhold the dose and inform the client of this. This is the desirable course of action. However, 32 per cent of pharmacists said they would provide the usual dose, 16 per cent would dispense a reduced dose without the client knowing and nine per cent said they would blind the dose with a placebo. Only two per cent of the pharmacists indicated that they would breathalyse an intoxicated client.

Pharmacists who withheld the methadone dose were more likely to inform the prescriber (74 per cent) than pharmacists who dispensed the usual or modified dose. In a focus group, the reasons for dispensing to an intoxicated client were categorized as follows:
- insufficient communication between prescriber and pharmacist
- downplaying the risk of toxicity
- personal beliefs and values
- fear of what the client would do if dose refused
- difficulty in recognizing intoxication and lack of education and training.

Further, Koutroulis et al.'s survey suggested that pharmacists who had more than 10 methadone clients were more likely to provide the usual methadone dose than pharmacists with 10 or fewer clients.

EDUCATIONAL OFFERINGS

> Many physicians and pharmacists don't think they see addicts in their practice. The reality is they probably are treating them for other disorders, but the patient just hasn't been identified as an addict. This also means that dependence treatment needs to become part of regular pharmacy practice as well.
> —Open discussion, physicians and pharmacists
> (Raisch et al., 2005)

The panel recommends that:
16. All pharmacy students receive education on substance abuse, including opioid dependence, its treatment and practical intervention strategies, in their undergraduate curriculum. [IV]

Future pharmacists need to be adequately educated on substance use so that they are prepared upon graduation to care for patients with substance abuse disorders. In particular, opioid dependence and its treatment should be required components in the curriculum. Pharmacists who have had education in this area are likely to feel more comfortable providing pharmaceutical care to this group of clients.

Currently there are two faculties of pharmacy in Ontario, at the University of Toronto and at the University of Waterloo. The Waterloo faculty initiated their program in January 2009; therefore, their plans for curriculum on substance abuse education are still in the development phase.

At Toronto's Faculty of Pharmacy, pharmacy students receive a rigorous scientific and clinical education over four years but receive little or no education on substance abuse and its treatment. Since the early 1990s, an elective fourth-year problem-based course has been offered (Busto et al., 1994). This course has one 2-hour segment on opioid abuse and treatment. It includes a didactic component, as well as an MMT client interview and discussion of stigma and attitudes. The course is elective and only a small proportion of the fourth-year class has taken this course offering.

Over the last five years enrolment in this elective has increased from 9.7 per cent of the class (13/134 students) in 2003–2004 to 34.2 per cent of the class (79/231 students) in 2008–2009 (personal communication, Dr. B. Sproule, April 29, 2009). Clearly, most future pharmacists have no exposure to substance use, opioid dependence and treatment with methadone.

The lack of specific undergraduate educational activities about substance abuse results in a missed opportunity to positively influence the knowledge, skills and attitudes of future pharmacists in this area.

As the most accessible of all health care professionals, pharmacists have an important role to play to help prevent and treat substance abuse disorders in their clients (Tommasello, 2004). Preparation for this role should begin in the undergraduate pharmacy training.

Experiential learning and other innovative teaching methods, for example, involving real patients (or simulated cases), audiovisual vignettes or other online modules may enhance pharmacy students' understanding of substance dependence issues and attitudes.

One college of pharmacy in the United States, in addition to a required substance abuse course, offers an elective to illustrate addiction recovery principles. Students taking the elective are asked to give up a habit that is causing them problems for six weeks and they meet weekly to discuss the addiction recovery process. This course has been offered for 15 years and 50 per cent of the substance abuse course students are enrolled (Baldwin, 2008).

FROM THE CLIENT CONSULTATION INTERVIEWS

CLIENTS' NEED FOR PHARMACEUTICAL CARE

"I would have liked to know more about methadone before I started. It would have helped me make a better decision. You shouldn't just tell a sick person 'this will make you better.'"

"There has been a lack of care and communication and confusion with my HIV meds. The methadone wasn't holding me due to medication interactions."

"I felt sick for weeks and didn't know it was because my dose was too high."

The panel recommends that:
17. Professional organizations, addiction and mental health agencies and pharmacists' employers promote the development of, and provide encouragement for all practising pharmacists to participate in, educational events on substance abuse and opioid dependence, including the growing problem of prescription opioid abuse. [III]

Most pharmacists receive little training on opioid dependence and treatment in their undergraduate experience, and it is important that all pharmacists further their knowledge in this area, even if they are not yet providing MMT services. There are indications that abuse and dependence on prescription opioids is increasing in Ontario and Canada. There was an increased number of patients addicted to prescription opioids entering the CAMH methadone maintenance program following the rapid expansion in the availability of MMT in Ontario in the 1990s (Brands et al., 2002; Brands et al., 2000). More recently, the number of individuals seeking detoxification treatment from controlled-release oxycodone at CAMH has also increased significantly (Sproule et al., 2009). In addition, in a cohort study of illicit opioid users, the proportion using prescription opioids increased from the year 2002 to 2005, with regional differences noted across Canada (Fischer et al., 2006). Pharmacists need to increase their knowledge base in prescription opioid addiction, particularly to understand the difference between addiction and physical dependence. Continuing education programs on pain treatment rarely (or inadequately) discuss the issue of opioid abuse and dependence.

A survey in British Columbia of 257 pharmacists (Cohen & McCormick, 2008) found that a slight majority reported training on how to identify signs of prescription drug misuse or abuse. This training was more common in younger pharmacists. The mean amount of training was 13.6 hours. Many pharmacists learned to identify prescription drug misuse through personal experience: they detected multi-doctoring using the provincial PharmaNet prescription drug profile or by recognizing early refills of prescriptions. Most intervened by calling the physician to confirm prescriptions or by confronting the customer directly. The primary reason they gave for not intervening was concern over how the customer might react (i.e., they were afraid that the client would be confrontational or they feared for their own safety). Pharmacists recommended additional training on prescription drug misuse.

Jones et al. (2005) surveyed 42 community pharmacists in Wales and found that at one month after a structured educational evening event there was little maintained change in attitudes. This suggests that changing attitudes is a long-term process. There is a need for reinforcing changes through continuing education.

Practising pharmacists (484) in Florida were surveyed while attending continuing education programs (Lafferty et al., 2006). Of the respondents, 67.5 per cent reported participating in two or fewer hours of addiction/substance abuse education in pharmacy school and 29.2 per cent said they had received no addiction education. Pharmacists who had more education counselled clients more frequently and felt more confident in dealing with substance abuse clients. Of those surveyed, 53 per cent reported they had never referred a patient to substance abuse treatment in their whole career.

Brooks et al. (2001) conducted a survey in the United States of 556 pharmacists, comparing those who had taken training in addiction treatment to those who had not, and found that those who had taken training would more likely refer clients to community resources and be more involved in working with their chemically dependent clients.

The panel recommends that:

18. The Ontario College of Pharmacists revise the current requirements for pharmacies providing MMT services to mandate earlier training to promote safety. The designated manager and one pharmacist must complete the training within six months of starting to dispense methadone. [IV]

19. CAMH or another approved provider of methadone training develop a brief electronic document (e.g., one page) outlining the key safety features of providing MMT services that can be made available for immediate use by pharmacies initiating MMT services. [IV]

20. CAMH produce an electronic version of its most recent pharmacist's guide to methadone maintenance treatment that can be purchased on-line and downloaded immediately so that pharmacies initiating MMT services can access it without delay. [IV]

21. CAMH make the online component of its Opioid Dependence Treatment Course available immediately upon enrolment to pharmacists new to providing MMT services, with the stipulation that these pharmacists attend the workshop component within six months of beginning the course. [IV]

22. CAMH or another approved provider of methadone training monitor and respond to waiting lists for training programs by, for example, offering

the training more frequently or by exploring other delivery methods, such as webinars or video conferencing, to help meet the needs of pharmacists in remote areas. [IV]

Since undergraduate training on substance abuse and opioid dependence is lacking, most pharmacists do not have an adequate knowledge base from which to provide MMT services safely.

Having the most essential knowledge and references easily accessible and as early as possible will help facilitate pharmacies starting a methadone service and assist those who are deciding whether to provide MMT.

The online component of the CAMH Opiate Dependence Treatment Interprofessional Education Program would provide a good introduction to providing service, and a brief methadone information sheet would complement this program. The methadone information sheet could include some of the key points in providing MMT service, for example, observing dosing, diluting dose in orange drink, identifying the client, assessing the client for intoxication and informing the prescriber of missed doses.

Having a current version of the CAMH *Pharmacist's Guide* available in a downloadable format would enable pharmacists to have this mandatory reference as soon as they need it. The other two references pharmacists dispensing methadone require, the CPSO *Methadone Maintenance Guidelines* and the OCP *Policy for Dispensing Methadone*, are currently available electronically.

The panel recommends that:
23. The Ontario College of Pharmacists and providers of methadone training collaborate on ongoing training requirements based on needs identified during the College's pharmacy inspection process. [IV]

The Ontario College of Pharmacists undertakes regular inspections of community pharmacy practice in the province. Practice issues related to methadone service provision identified during these inspections could be shared with educational service providers for consideration in future training initiatives. This would be an effective mechanism for updating methadone training to reflect current practice issues in the field.

The panel recommends that:
24. CAMH or another approved provider of methadone education deliver methadone training in a manner consistent with interprofessional education principles. [IV]

Since MMT practice is best delivered in a collaborative manner (Health Canada, 2002), a multidisciplinary approach in education will prepare pharmacists to work effectively with other health professionals as a team.

The panel recommends that:
25. The Ontario College of Pharmacists and community colleges providing pharmacy technician training develop core competency requirements for regulated pharmacy technicians providing M MT services. [IV]

Pharmacy technicians are important members of the pharmacy team. They may be involved with preparing and dispensing methadone, and interact with MMT clients in the pharmacy. Core competencies should be developed and educational programs designed to optimize the role of pharmacy technicians in the safe delivery of methadone services. This issue may be particularly important in view of the new regulated status for pharmacy technicians that will be implemented soon in Ontario, where pharmacy technicians will be able to take more responsibility for dispensing.

The panel recommends that:
26. CAMH or another approved provider of methadone education undertake a needs assessment of pharmacists who have participated in the initial M MT training, and then use this information to develop an updated or advanced MMT course for pharmacists. [IV]

27. Professional pharmacy organizations, the Ontario College of Pharmacists, pharmacy managers/owners and hospital pharmacy directors encourage pharmacists to take courses on motivational interviewing, intervention strategies to use with difficult patients, and concurrent disorders, to enhance pharmacists' skills in dealing with opioid-dependent clients. [IV]

Pharmacists who are already in MMT practice and have taken initial MMT training may wish to update and improve their skills. Since pharmacist training is recommended by the Ontario College of Pharmacists every five years, a new, higher level course would meet the needs of this experienced group of providers. Pharmacists who have taken initial MMT training should be surveyed for their input about topics to include within this higher level course. This advanced training could include, for example, methadone use in pregnancy, in patients with concurrent disorders (e.g., pain, psychiatric disorders, HIV) and in other special populations.

Any interaction with a client has therapeutic potential. Pharmacists using motivational techniques in their interactions with clients may enhance clients' treatment. The issue of dealing with difficult, demanding clients has been identified by pharmacists as an area in which they would like more training (Cohen & McCormick, 2008). Training in de-escalation techniques to avoid potentially unsafe interactions could help pharmacists achieve greater satisfaction in their practice, as well as improve client outcomes.

The panel recommends that:
28. Drug information service providers ensure that staff is trained on and familiar with common issues in MMT treatment and have a mechanism to refer to experts when necessary. [IV]

Pharmacies must subscribe to a drug information provider service. The staff at the drug information provider should be able to respond to general questions on MMT and substance abuse. To do this they would require training in MMT to understand the patient safety issues and relevant guidelines. For more complex questions, the drug information service should have an arrangement with expert service providers to assist in consultation.

The panel recommends that:
29. Professional pharmacy organizations develop a mechanism in conjunction with the Ontario College of Pharmacists to ensure that pharmacists dispensing methadone are informed in a timely fashion of new educational resources available. [IV]

A timely direct communication via e-mail from the Ontario College of Pharmacists, the Ontario Pharmacists' Association or another professional pharmacy organization is recommended when any new methadone-related item is posted on the website of either the OCP or the CPSO.

The panel recommends that:

30. Professional pharmacy organizations, CAMH and funding agencies develop a mentorship program to link new methadone service providers with experienced providers. [IV]

31. Professional pharmacy organizations and CAMH promote the CAMH Addiction Clinical Consultation Service to pharmacists providing MMT services. [IV]

The Addiction Clinical Consultation Service (ACCS) is a service provided by CAMH. It is designed to serve health and social service professionals, including pharmacists, who have client-specific questions related to substance abuse. The ACCS is not designed to deal with health emergencies or immediate or legal issues. The health care worker calls a central phone number and, depending on the question, ACCS may provide referral to a consultant team member (physician, therapist/counsellor or pharmacist) who will communicate with the health care worker within four hours. Awareness of the service should be promoted to support pharmacists providing methadone services.

Research in MMT pharmacy practice

There is a significant lack of research on pharmacy services in MMT in Ontario. Most pharmacy-based research available consists of descriptive survey-type studies conducted in other countries.

Some areas for future research have already been recommended in earlier sections. In "Accessibility of MMT pharmacy services," the panel recommended that pharmacists, particularly those in under-serviced areas, be surveyed for their views and concerns about participation in MMT programs, that the efficacy of offering incentives to encourage them to provide MMT services be investigated and that fair and equitable payment models for pharmacy MMT services be explored and evaluated (recommendations 10, 11 and 12, respectively).

In addition to these recommendations, research focusing on the impact of pharmacy services on client outcomes is much in need.

The panel recommends that:

32. Scientists in Ontario develop a research program to investigate all aspects of pharmacy practice in MMT, including:

a. the effectiveness of different models of care (including those with pharmacists in community pharmacies and in clinic settings)

b. the impact of pharmacist interventions on client outcomes

c. pharmacoeconomic implications

d. factors that could affect community pharmacy capacity to accommodate MMT clients

e. possible ways to increase access to methadone pharmacy services in remote areas. [IV]

33. Investigators study the impact of educational initiatives on patient outcomes. [IV]

Conclusion:
Beyond the recommendations

Beyond the scope of this document, there are other topics related to methadone and the treatment of opioid dependence that are important and require future consideration. In particular, pharmacists providing methadone services for patients with pain outside an addiction context still require knowledge of methadone's unique pharmacology, to protect against the risk of overdose, and knowledge of its potential for abuse, to protect against the risk of diversion. Also, buprenorphine is emerging in Ontario as an alternative medication for the treatment of opioid dependence.

Buprenorphine has some unique pharmacological properties that positively impact clinical care (e.g., improved safety profile, potential for less than daily dosing). However, pharmacists must also understand its pharmacology to appropriately start a client on buprenorphine (i.e., induction strategies). This drug also has a risk for diversion. Clinical practice guidelines for buprenorphine are not yet available in Ontario. Future best practice documents for the treatment of opioid dependence should include both methadone and buprenorphine.

The purpose of this guide is to provide recommendations for enhancing pharmacy services in methadone maintenance treatment in Ontario at the pharmacy and system level. It addresses issues beyond the individual pharmacist, making recommendations related to the pharmacy environment, pharmacist education programs, accessibility of pharmacy services and research needs. Consideration and adoption of these recommendations by pharmacy managers, corporate executives, the Ontario College of Pharmacists, pharmacy educational institutions, research scientists, professional pharmacy organizations and the government would provide significant support to pharmacists to provide best practice methadone services, with the goal of enhancing safety and improving therapeutic outcomes for clients in MMT. The results of needed pharmacy practice–based research would help inform future best practice guides for pharmacists providing service for opioid-dependent clients.

REFERENCES

American Society of Health-System Pharmacists. (2003). ASHP statement on the pharmacist's role in substance abuse prevention, education, and assistance. *American Journal of Health-System Pharmacy, 60* (19), 1995–1998.

Anstice, S., Strike, C.J. & Brands, B. (2009). Supervised methadone consumption: Client issues and stigma. *Substance Use & Misuse, 44* (6), 794–808.

Baldwin, J.N. (2008). A guided abstinence experience to illustrate addiction recovery principles. *American Journal of Pharmaceutical Education, 72* (4), 78.

Berbatis, C., Sunderland, V.B. & Bulsara, M. (2003). The services provided by community pharmacists to prevent, minimize and manage drug misuse: An international perspective. In J. Sheridan & J. Strang (Eds.), *Drug Misuse and Community Pharmacy* (pp. 73–84). London, UK: Taylor & Francis.

Bond, C. (Ed.). (2000). *Evidence-based Pharmacy.* London, UK: Pharmaceutical Press.

Brands, B., Blake, J. & Marsh, D. (2002). Changing patient characteristics with increased methadone maintenance availability. *Drug & Alcohol Dependence, 66* (1), 11–20.

Brands, J., Brands, B. & Marsh, D. (2000). The expansion of methadone prescribing in Ontario, 1996–1997. *Addiction Research & Theory, 8* (5), 485–496.

Brooks, V., Brock, T. & Ahn, J. (2001). Do training programs work? An assessment of pharmacists' activities in the field of chemical dependency. *Journal of Drug Education, 31* (2), 153–169.

Budd, G. & McClelland, M. (2006, July). Methadone maintenance program overview. College of Pharmacists of British Columbia. Available: www.bcpharmacists.org/library/H-Resources/H-4_Pharmacy_Resources/5058-Methadone_Maintenance_Program_Overview.pdf. Accessed May 27, 2009.

Busto, U., Knight, K., Janececk, E., Isaac, P. & Parker, K. (1994). A problem-based learning course for pharmacy students on alcohol and psychoactive substance abuse disorders. *American Journal of Pharmaceutical Education, 58* (1), 55–60.

Canadian Patient Safety Institute. (2008). Safer Healthcare Now! Reducing Harm, Improving Healthcare, Protecting Canadians. Available: www.saferhealthcarenow.ca. Accessed June 1, 2009.

Cohen, I.M. & McCormick, A.V. (2008). The role of pharmacists in the identification and prevention of prescription drug misuse. BC Centre for Social Responsibility. Available: www.bccsr.ca. Accessed June 1, 2009.

Collège des médecins du Québec & Ordre des pharmaciens du Québec. (2000). *Clinical Practice Guidelines: The Use of Methadone in the Treatment of Opioid Addiction.* Quebec City: Author.

College of Pharmacists of British Columbia. (2007). *Pharmacy Methadone Maintenance Guide.* Vancouver: Author.

College of Physicians and Surgeons of Ontario (CPSO). (2005). *Methadone Maintenance Guidelines*. Toronto: Author.

Curnan, V., Ungar, T. & Pauzé, E. (2006, February). *Strengthening Collaboration Through Interprofessional Education: A Resource for Collaborative Mental Health Care Educators*. Mississauga, ON: Canadian Collaborative Mental Health Initiative. Available: www.ccmhi.ca. Accessed May 27, 2009.

Drucker, E., Rice, S., Ganse, G., Kegley, J., Bosnuck, K. & Tuchman, E. (2007). The Lancaster office based opiate treatment program: A case study and prototype for community physicians and pharmacists providing methadone maintenance treatment in the United States. *Addictive Disorders & Their Treatment, 6* (3), 121–135.

First Canadian Health (FCH) on behalf of Health Canada. Refusal to dispense program for British Columbia. (2007, Spring). *Non-Insured Health Benefits (NHIB) Newsletter for Pharmacy Providers*. Available: www.hc-sc.gc.ca/fniah-spnia/pubs/nihb-ssna/_drug-med/2007-news -spring-bull-print/index-eng.php. Accessed May 29, 2009.

Fischer, B., Rehm, J., Patra, J. & Cruz, M.F. (2006). Changes in illicit opioid use across Canada. *Canadian Medical Association Journal, 175* (11), 1385.

Gastelurrutia, M.A., Faus, M.J. & Fernandez-Llimos, F. (2005). Providing patient care in community pharmacies in Spain. *The Annals of Pharmacotherapy, 39* (12), 2105–2110.

Glasgow City Council (2008, June 6). Methadone and the Shared Care Programme. Available: www.glasgow.gov.uk/en/Residents/Care_Support/Drugs_Alcohol/Information/ Whatisthemethadoneprogramme/. Accessed May 27, 2009.

Graham, A., Pfeifer, J., Trumble, J. & Nelson, E. (1999). A pilot project: Continuing education for pharmacists on substance abuse prevention. *Substance Abuse, 20* (1), 33–43.

Hart, W.A. (2007). *Report of the Methadone Maintenance Treatment Practices Task Force*. Toronto: Ontario Ministry of Health and Long-Term Care.

Health Canada. (2002). *Best Practices: Methadone Maintenance Treatment*. Ottawa: Minister of Public Works and Government Services.

HealthForceOntario (2007). *Interprofessional Care: A Blueprint for Action in Ontario*. Toronto: Author.

Isaac, P., Kalvik, A., Brands, J. & Janecek, E. (Eds.). *Methadone Maintenance: A Pharmacist's Guide to Treatment. Second Edition*. Toronto: CAMH, 2004.

Jones, L., Edge, J. & Love, A. (2005). The effect of educational intervention on pharmacists' attitudes to substance misusers. *Journal of Substance Use, 10* (5), 285–292.

Keene, J., Ahmed, S., Fenley, S. & Walker, M. (2004). A qualitative study of a successful shared care project for heroin users: The Berkshire Four Way Agreement. *International Journal of Drug Policy, 15* (3), 196–201.

Koutroulis, G.Y., Kutin, J.J., Ugoni, A.M., Odgers, P., Muhleisen, P., Ezard, N. et al. (2000). Pharmacists' provision of methadone to intoxicated clients in community pharmacies, Victoria, Australia. *Drug and Alcohol Review, 19* (3), 299–308.

Kroger, E., Moisan, J. & Gregoire, J.P. (2000). Billing for cognitive services: Understanding Quebec pharmacists' behavior. *The Annals of Pharmacotherapy, 34* (3), 309–316.

Lafferty, L., Hunter, T.S. & Marsh, W.A. (2006). Knowledge, attitudes and practices of pharmacists concerning prescription drug abuse. *Journal of Psychoactive Drugs, 38* (3), 229–232.

Lawrie, T., Matheson, C., Bond, C.M. & Roberts, K. (2004). Pharmacy customers' views and experiences of using pharmacies which provide drug misuse services. *Drug and Alcohol Review, 23* (2), 195–202.

Lawrinson, P., Roche, A., Terao, H. & Le, P.P. (2008). Dispensing opioid substitution treatment: Practices, attitudes and intentions of community-based pharmacists. *Drug and Alcohol Review, 27* (1), 47–53.

Lea, T., Sheridan, J. & Winstock, A. (2008). Consumer satisfaction with opioid treatment services at community pharmacies in Australia. *Pharmacy World & Science, 30* (6), 940–946.

Li, A. (1996, June). *Evaluation of the Community Pharmacist's Role in Dispensing Methadone.* A report submitted to the Joint Residency Committee of the Clinical Research and Treatment Institute, Addiction Research Foundation and the Faculty of Pharmacy, University of Toronto, in partial fulfilment of its requirement for the certificate of the Canadian Hospital Pharmacy Residency Programme. Toronto: Addiction Research Foundation.

Luger, L., Bathia, N., Alcorn, R. & Power, R. (2000). Involvement of community pharmacists in the care of drug misusers: Pharmacy-based supervision of methadone consumption. *International Journal on Drug Policy, 11* (3), 227–234.

Mackie, C., Healy, A.M., Roberts, K. & Ryder, S. (2004). A comparison of community pharmacy methadone services between Dublin and Glasgow: (1) Extent of service provision in 1997/1998 and views of pharmacists on existing provision and future service developments. *Journal of Substance Use, 9* (5), 235–251.

Matheson, C. (2003). Drug users and pharmacists: The client perspective. In J. Sheridan & J. Strang (Eds.), *Drug Misuse and Community Pharmacy* (pp. 85–96). London, UK: Taylor & Francis.

Matheson, C., Bond, C.M. & Hickey, F. (1999). Prescribing and dispensing for drug misusers in primary care: Current practice in Scotland. *Family Practice, 16* (4), 375–379.

Matheson, C., Bond, C.M. & Mollison, J. (1999). Attitudinal factors associated with community pharmacists' involvement in services for drug misusers. *Addiction, 94* (9), 1349–1359.

Matheson, C., Bond, C.M. & Pitcairn, J. (2002). Community pharmacy services for drug misusers in Scotland: What difference does 5 years make? *Addiction, 97* (11), 1405–1411.

Matheson, C., Bond, C.M. & Tinelli, M. (2007). Community pharmacy harm reduction services for drug misusers: National service delivery and professional attitude development over a decade in Scotland. *Journal of Public Health (Oxford, England), 29* (4), 350–357.

Merrill, J.O., Jackson, T.R., Schulman, B.A., Saxon, A.J., Awan, A., Kapitan, S. et al. (2005). Methadone medical maintenance in primary care: An implementation evaluation. *Journal of General Internal Medicine, 20* (4), 344–349.

Myers, T., Cockerill, R., Worthington, C., Millson, M. & Rankin, J. (1998). Community pharmacist perspectives on HIV/AIDS and interventions for injection drug users in Canada. *AIDS Care, 10* (6), 689–700.

Neale, J. (1998). Drug users' views of drug service providers. *Health & Social Care in the Community, 6* (5), 308–317.

New Brunswick Addiction Services. (2005). *Methadone Maintenance Treatment Guidelines.* Fredericton: Author.

Nielsen, S., Dietze, P., Dunlop, A., Muhleisen, P., Lee, N. & Taylor, D. (2007). Buprenorphine supply by community pharmacists in Victoria, Australia: Perceptions, experiences and key issues identified. *Drug and Alcohol Review, 26* (2), 143–151.

Ontario College of Pharmacists (OCP). (September 1, 2006). *Policy for Dispensing Methadone.* Toronto: Author. Available: http://www.ocpinfo.com/client/ocp/OCPHome.nsf/object/ Methadone_Policy_06/$file/Methadone_Policy_06.pdf. Accessed May 27, 2009.

Ontario College of Pharmacists. (OCP). (2008). Coroner's report: Combined toxic effects of methadone and ethanol. *Pharmacy Connection,* (March/April), 38–39.

Peterson, G.M. (1999). Drug misuse and harm reduction: Pharmacy's magnificent contribution, but at what cost? *Journal of Clinical Pharmacy and Therapeutics, 24* (3), 165–169.

Peterson, G.M., Northeast, S., Jackson, S.L. & Fitzmaurice, K.D. (2007). Harm minimization strategies: Opinions of health professionals in rural and remote Australia. *Journal of Clinical Pharmacy and Therapeutics, 32* (5), 497–504.

Raisch, D.W., Fudala, P.J., Saxon, A.J., Walsh, R., Casadonte, P., Ling, W. et al. (2005). Pharmacists' and technicians' perceptions and attitudes toward dispensing buprenorphine/naloxone to patients with opioid dependence. *Journal of the American Pharmaceutical Association (2003), 45* (1), 23–32.

Roberts, K., Murray, H. & Gilmour, R. (2007). What's the problem? Why do some pharmacists provide services to drug users and others won't? *Journal of Substance Use, 12* (1), 13–25.

Samitca, S., Huissoud, T., Jeannin, A. & Dubois-Arber, F. (2007). The role of pharmacies in the care of drug users: What has changed in ten years. The case of a Swiss region. *European Addiction Research, 13,* (1), 50–56.

Shared Care Monitoring Group. (2005, September). *Guidelines for Supervised Consumption of Methadone.* East Yorkshire, UK: NHS East Yorkshire and Wolds & Coast Primary Care Trusts. Available: www.erypct.nhs.uk/upload/HERHIS/East%20Riding%20PCTs/Document%20Store/ Policies/CP%2037%20Supervised%20Consumption.pdf. Accessed May 27, 2009.

Sheridan, J. & Barber, N. (1997). Drug misuse and HIV prevention: Attitudes and practices of community pharmacists with respect to two London family health service authorities. *Addiction Research, 15* (1), 11–21.

Sheridan, J., Manning, V., Ridge, G., Mayet, S. & Strang, J. (2007). Community pharmacies and the provision of opioid substitution services for drug misusers: Changes in activity and attitudes of community pharmacists across England 1995–2005. *Addiction, 102* (11), 1824–1830.

Sheridan, J. & Strang, J. Eds. (2003). *Drug Misuse and Community Pharmacy.* London, UK: Taylor & Francis.

Sproule, B.A., Brands, B., Li, S., & Catz-Biro, L. (2009). Changing patterns in opioid addiction: Characterizing users of oxycodone and other opioids. *Canadian Family Physician, 55* (1), 68–69.e5.

Sutcliffe, N. (2009). Profile of the relief pharmacist. *Pharmacy Connection* (March/April), 6–7.

Tommasello, A.C. (2004). Substance abuse and pharmacy practice: What the community pharmacist needs to know about drug abuse and dependence. *Harm Reduction Journal, 1* (1), 3.

Tuchman, E. (2008). A model-guided process evaluation: Office-based prescribing and pharmacy dispensing of methadone. *Evaluation and Program Planning, 31* (4), 376–381.

Tuchman, E., Bonuck, K., Tommasello, A. & Drucker, E. (2003). Office based methadone treatment: A role for community pharmacists. *Addictive Disorders & Their Treatment, 2* (3), 91–96.

RESOURCES

For more information on CAMH publications, educational resources and training programs, please visit www.camh.net and follow the links.

The following is a select list of resources from CAMH.

Methadone Saves Lives
The MethadoneSavesLives.ca website is a portal to a comprehensive range of information about opioid dependence and treatment that is written accessibly for clients and care providers. It provides the facts that both professionals and people living with opioid drug problems (and their family and friends) need to make informed decisions about MMT.

The site contains information about:
- where to find help and an MMT program
- different types of opioid drugs, including the "Straight Talk" and "Do You Know" pamphlet series
- online tutorials about addiction
- how to order or download copies of CAMH publications, such as the *Methadone Maintenance Treatment: Client Handbook* and *Methadone Maintenance Treatment: A Community Planning Guide*
- how to order other educational materials such as the *Prescription for Addiction* DVD and user's guide.

The site also contains information on CAMH's Opiate Dependence Treatment Interprofessional Education Program, which prepares physicians, pharmacists, nurses, counsellors and case managers to provide a comprehensive range of services for people with opioid dependence.

To explore the site, go to www.MethadoneSavesLives.ca.

Methadone Maintenance Treatment: A Community Planning Guide
Written by Mark Erdelyan, Senior Program Consultant, CAMH Windsor

This manual offers guidance to communities on how to educate community members about the benefits of MMT and to develop and integrate effective treatment services. It reviews the stages of:
• establishing a community working group
• engaging the community, and
• planning, implementing and evaluating an MMT program.

The resource provides practical suggestions on how to build public support and increase acceptance of those struggling with opioid dependence, through raising community awareness and acceptance of MMT services.

For more information, search Education and Courses on www.camh.net.

Methadone Maintenance Treatment: Best Practices in Case Management
Kate Tschakovsky, MSW, RSW, Project Co-ordinator, OpiATE Project, CAMH

The first evidence-based guide written for case managers working with MMT clients in Ontario, this book describes the case manager's roles of co-ordination, counselling and advocacy at the hub of a circle of collaborative, professional care. It makes recommendations about what clinicians, the agencies they work for, policy-makers and funding bodies need to do to achieve and support best practice in case management. Many composite case studies, practice points and clients' quotations illustrate the issues and how best practices apply in different clinical scenarios.

For more information, search Education and Courses on www.camh.net.